BREAKING FREE:

Conquer Your Cravings and End Binge Eating.

BY

Lizzy F. Grant

TABLE OF CONTENTS

Chapter One

Definition: What exactly is Binge Eating Disorder?

Introduction

One kind of feeding and eating disorder that is currently formally recognized is binge eating disorder (BED). It can result in further diet-related health issues like diabetes and high cholesterol, and it affects approximately 2% of the world's population. Feeding and eating disorders are not solely about food, which is why they are classified as psychiatric disorders. People usually develop them to cope with a deeper issue or another psychological condition, such as anxiety or depression.

Do you find yourself having binge-eating episodes? Do you eat a lot of food and then feel guilty or ashamed about it? Do you find yourself in a binge-eating cycle? If this is the case, you may be suffering from a binge eating disorder. In this book, several of your questions will be answered, such as "Why do I binge eat? How can I stop binge-eating? What are the necessary treatments for binge eating? The book examines the symptoms, causes, and health risks associated with BED, as well as how to seek help and support in order to overcome it. The book suggests a self-help approach to binge eating disorder treatment as well as suggestive therapeutic assistance.

Definition:

What Exactly Is Binge Eating Disorder? (BED)

Binge eating is defined as eating a large amount of food in a short period of time, usually as part of an eating disorder. It is more than just feeling 'stuffed' or overeating on occasion. Binge eating disorder causes binges to become a regular occurrence. BED is characterized by repeated episodes of uncontrollable consumption of unusually large amounts of food in a short period of time. Feelings of guilt, shame, and psychological distress accompany these episodes. BED is defined by recurrent episodes of uncontrollable food eating that occur over a short period of time and in exceptionally large quantities. These events are accompanied by feelings of guilt, shame, and psychological discomfort.

The duration of a binge-eating episode might range from much less to much more than an hour. There are times when binge eating is a deliberate activity and times when it is not. A quarter of binges exceed 2,000 calories, with most involving more than 1,000 calories ingested. The key distinction between binge eating and overeating is a loss of control, and binge eating is when someone eats in a way that makes him feel like he has no control over what or how much he is eating or that he simply cannot stop.

People frequently would mention that they had struggled with other types of problems like alcohol or drug problems, as well as other problems where one felt like that level of loss of control, when we discussed binge eating disorder with them, which was one of the early things we did when we were trying to understand more about this new diagnosis. A binge eating disorder must also exhibit additional traits, such as genuine concern over food. It's possible for someone to think, "I ate a little more ice cream than I planned to." That was a little out of hand, I believe, but some claim that despite their distress, they continue to eat until they are filled, consume food when they are not even hungry, or conceal the signs of their binge eating. Binge eating disorder is a relapsing disorder that occurs in fits and starts.

People with binge eating disorders will typically go through cycles of out-of-control bingeing and then pulling it together and dieting to control the behavior. At the same time, overcontrol may be unsustainable over a period of time. It is possible to lose control again and go back to binge eating, and when those kinds of criteria are invoked, a much smaller percentage of people actually meet the criteria for this binge eating disorder.

Chapter Two

Symptoms of Binge Eating

Three or more of the following symptoms must be present for a healthcare professional to diagnose BED: 1. An Unexpected Meal: Whether you have this disease or not, it is always important to plan your meals. To begin with, it will assist you in maintaining a healthy diet. Whatever happens, you will stay on track. Similarly, without a routine, binge eaters struggle to control their food intake. They will binge for one meal and then, most likely, not eat for several hours. Their habits contribute to their overeating in this way.

2. Binge eating is not synonymous with bulimia.

Someone who binges will feel uncomfortable. Bulimia is a disease in which someone vomits to relieve the discomfort caused by binge-eating. Binge eating causes harm to the body, but bulimia causes severe harm. Bulimia does not affect every binge eater.

3. Getting obsessed in a short time

One of the most detrimental effects of binge-eating is obesity. A normal weight increase should not be mistaken for obesity. Throughout their lives, many people, especially women, endure typical weight fluctuations. Obesity is a medical disease that has a wide range of detrimental effects on one's health. Obesity increases the risk of cardiovascular conditions like diabetes, cancer, and chronic pain. To avoid overeating, eat more nutrient-dense foods to fill you up and boost your metabolism.

4. Total Lack of Self-Control

We are all aware that we should eat only when we are hungry. We sometimes choose to ignore this. The sensation of being full is satisfying and can improve any situation. It is critical to understand when and how to say "enough is enough" to food. It is not a good idea to keep eating after you are full. This is essential if you want to heal your relationship with food. Consider it a habit similar to turning off the lights or putting shoes in the closet.

5. Emotional Health Problems

Overeating is as bad for the mind as it is for the body. Sadness, anger, or stress can all be triggers for this disorder. Many people find comfort in food, which leads to bingeing. You may feel good while eating, but once you stop, the negative emotions return. After a while, you will feel everything you have been avoiding all over again. Aside from food, try to find outlets that make you happy. Experiment with new sports, hobbies, and classes. You can also try to form new relationships or strengthen existing ones.

6. You are not chewing your food

It takes our bodies twenty minutes to recognize that they are full. If we eat too quickly, this will not happen, and we will continue to overeat. Sit down and get comfortable when you're having a meal. Take it easy. Chew your food more thoroughly than usual, as this aids both the digestive process and the sensation of fullness.

7. Feeling Emotionally Overwhelmed.

This disease can elicit a wide range of emotions. When someone binges, they may experience a rush of excitement. They may be disgusted when the bingeing period is over. Overeating has an impact on the brain as well as the body. Having a difficult time controlling emotions is just one of its consequences. Having said that, we can classify this condition as a mental disorder as well. It creates an endless cycle. We will seek comfort in food again as a result of our feelings of guilt and disappointment. The feeling of helplessness in breaking free from this cycle can be overwhelming.

8. Separating Yourself

Feelings of shame are frequently associated with binge eating. Someone may find themselves eating alone because they are afraid of being judged by others. Trying to keep this disease hidden will only make matters worse. Keeping yourself isolated from your friends and family is counterproductive. Instead, try to communicate with them. They can provide you with the assistance you require, and your problem will be resolved quickly.

9. Private Dining:

Binge eaters frequently keep their food hidden from others. They will eat them if they are left alone. Finding a peaceful place to eat becomes an important part of the ritual. Binge eaters have a habit of hoarding food. This is consistent with their proclivity for isolation.

To summarize, binge eating occurs when you do the following:

i.   Eating much faster than usual until uncomfortably full; eating large amounts without feeling hungry;

ii.   Eating alone due to feelings of embarrassment and shame, guilt or disgust with oneself

iii. feeling depressed or extremely guilty afterward.

iv.   Binge eating is not connected with bulimia nervosa-like repetitive use of inappropriate compensatory behaviours (e.g., cleansing), and it does not occur only during the course of bulimia nervosa or anorexia nervosa.

5. Binge eating is associated with significant distress.

6. Binge eating occurs at least once a week, on average, for three months.

10.   Lying and Deceiving Others: When you separate yourself from others, you may appear to them to be quite normal. But you are aware that you are struggling on the inside. Pretending to have a normal eating schedule is harmful to this disease. However, things could get worse. Your friends have no idea you are dealing with a major problem on a daily basis. It has the potential to grow into something much larger, causing even more problems than you already have.

Physical Symptoms of Binge Eating Disorder
  i. Weight fluctuations are noticeable, as are up-and-down stomach cramps and other non-specific gastrointestinal complaints (constipation, acid reflux, etc.).
  ii. Problems with concentration

This is not an exhaustive list of binge eating disorder symptoms. However, a licensed provider should be consulted to determine the diagnosis and treatment. People suffering from BED frequently express extreme dissatisfaction and distress about their eating habits, body shape, and weight. Even if they are not hungry, people with BED may consume a large amount of food in a short period of time. Emotional stress or de-stressing frequently plays a role and can lead to binge eating. A person may feel a sense of release or relief during a binge, but afterwards, they may feel shame or a loss of control.

Chapter Three

Causes of Binge Eating

Uncertainty exists about the causes of BED. Additionally, there is no single risk factor that promotes binge-eating; rather, a number of risk variables work together to do so.

i. Genetics: Dopamine, a brain chemical that's involved in sensations of reward and pleasure, may be more sensitive in people with BED. Additionally, there is compelling evidence that the condition is hereditary.

ii. Alterations in the brain: There are signs that people with BED may experience structural changes in the brain that affect how responsive they are to food and how well they can control themselves.

iii. Body Weight: Obesity affects about 50% of those with BED, and 25–50% of individuals undergoing weight loss surgery also have BED. Weight issues may both contribute to and be a symptom of the condition.

iv.   Gender: Women are more likely than men to experience BED. 3.6% of American women and 2.0% of American men have BED at some point in their lives. There may be underlying biological causes for this.

v.   Body Image: Many BED sufferers have a very poor perception of their bodies. Dieting, overeating, and body dissatisfaction all play a role in the disorder's emergence.

vi.   A Binge Meal: The first sign of the disorder, according to those who are affected, is frequently a history of binge eating. This involves binge eating in adolescence and childhood.

Other Psychiatric Issues:

About 80% of BED patients also experience at least one additional mental health condition, such as substance abuse, PTSD, anxiety, depression, bipolar disorder, or phobias.

Psychological Damage:

Stressful life events, including abuse, death, being far from family, and car accidents, are risk factors. Bullying in youngsters that is related to weight may also be a factor.

Binge-eating episodes can be caused by stress, dieting, negative body image concerns, the availability of food, boredom, or unpleasant thoughts about one's looks.

Chapter Four

Myths about Binge Eating

Myths around binge eating include the following:

First of all, it is well accepted that binge-eating disorders are complicated conditions impacted by a person's biology, environment, genetics, and family history.

Second, a common misperception is that binge eating disorder exclusively affects women and girls who identify as cisgender and who are white. However, research indicates that anyone can be affected by binge-eating problems. The misconception that eating disorders only affect specific individuals may keep some people from getting the care or diagnosis they need. This fallacy thereby fuels stigma and health inequalities within particular communities.

The idea that treating and preventing binge eating disorders requires nothing more complicated than loving oneself and leading a healthy lifestyle. Research indicates that binge eating disorder is a serious medical problem that may require several different types of treatment because of its intricate effects on a person's life and general health. Nutritional counselling, behavioural health modifications, therapy, and/or other treatments.

To give each person the best care possible for their particular needs, a combination of dietary advice, behavioural health adjustments, therapy, and/or other treatments may be used.

Speak with a medical expert to find out about treatment options if you or someone you know is suffering from eating disorder symptoms. Check out the treatment alternatives accessible in the media for these individuals if you're a provider seeking information on evidence-based treatment.

Chapter Five

Differences between a Binge Eating Disorder and Overeating

Even though there are clear distinctions between bingeing and overeating, some individuals are unclear which action they are engaging in.

i.   Binge eating disorder is not the same as overeating. It's common for people to overeat, and many do it on occasion.

ii.   Overeating is the act of consuming more food than normal for a particular purpose.

iii.   Holidays, festive dinners, and the presence of favoured foods are the times when overindulgence in food occurs most frequently.

iv.   Typically, overeating is described as consuming additional servings during a holiday meal or at a favoured restaurant. An individual may feel sick or guilty after overindulging, but these emotions normally subside and don't prompt significant lifestyle adjustments, such starting a low-calorie diet.

v.   On the other hand, binge eating entails periodic episodes of covert bingeing that function as a kind of self-soothing.

vi.   An example of binge eating would be overindulging over a holiday meal and then overindulging for a few months, at least once a week.

vii.   After eating, this person may feel ill and experience shame and guilt. Depression or yo-yo dieting may be brought on by these feelings.

viii.   On the other hand, people who obsessively binge eat could use food as their only coping mechanism for unpleasant emotions.

ix.   As a result, they often feel that their eating is uncontrollably excessive.

x.   They feel depressed, guilty, or embarrassed after eating and are preoccupied with food all the time.

xi.   On the other hand, overindulging in food can lead to feelings of fullness, even though the individual may not feel guilty about eating so much because they might not have the chance to eat as much in the coming weeks or months and may not be shame-obsessed.

Another scenario is the clinical condition known as binge eating disorder (BED), which is present in some overeaters.

BED sufferers overeat rapidly and compulsively, then feel guilty or embarrassed about it afterwards. And they do it regularly - for at least three months, at least once a week.

It's also important to realize that not everyone who overeats binges. You can spread out your meals throughout the day as an alternative to consuming a large amount of food at once. Rather than using it frequently, you might just use it infrequently when you're feeling depressed, lonely, or anxious.

Chapter Six

Health Issues Associated with Binge Eating Disorder

Binge eating disorder can affect anyone, regardless of gender, age, weight, or any other characteristic. Binge eating can be detected in people of any weight, but it is more common in overweight individuals, of whom two-thirds are considered clinically obese.

Similar to other eating disorders, binge eating disorder is a grave illness that can have negative consequences, including the following:

i.   Overweight or Obesity: These phrases describe excessive or inappropriate fat accumulation that is unhealthy. A body mass index (BMI) of 25 indicates overweight, whereas a BMI of more than 30 indicates obesity.

ii.   The BMI of an overweight person is at or above the 85th percentile but below the 95th percentile for children of the same age, and sex, which distinguishes them from obese people.

iii.   A child is deemed obese if their BMI is at or above the 95th percentile for children of the same age and sex. Binge eating usually results in weight gain.

Approximately two thirds of patients with the illness are overweight. You acquire weight when you eat a lot of food quickly without burning it off through exercise.

Many people who overeat also experience problems connected to their weight. This leads to low self-esteem, which may exacerbate binge eating. Furthermore, being obese or overweight can raise your chance of developing chronic health issues like:

     i.   Stopping breathing a lot during the night (sleep apnea).

     ii.   Specific types of cancer.

     iii.   Heart Condition: Being overweight puts more strain on your heart, making it work harder to pump blood to your body and lungs. Excess body fat, particularly around the belly, increases the risk of heart attacks and strokes.

iv.   High triglycerides;

v.   Diabetes type 2;

vi.   Arthritis; and

vii.   Elevated blood pressure;

viii.   Gallbladder illness

ix.   Mental health issues, particularly depression.

Chapter Seven

How to Identify Excess Weight

i.		Your clothes will start to feel tight. The readings on your bathroom scale will go up. To ascertain your body fat percentage, your physician will measure.

ii.		Body mass index, or BMI (weight to height ratio): The waist-hip ratio (WHR), which is used to quantify obesity, may also indicate other, more serious medical conditions.

iii.		The World Health Organization (WHO) defines abdominal obesity as having a body mass index (BMI) of more than 30.0 or a waist-hip ratio greater than 0.90 for males and 0.85 for females.

iv.		Your stomach's size is determined by placing a tape measure in the middle of your torso, above your hips (waist circumference).

v.		We'll test your blood pressure, blood sugar, and cholesterol because gaining weight can affect all of these parameters.

Chapter Eight:

Binge Eating Disorder Treatment

i. The first step in addressing binge eating is determining the cause of your overindulgence. This may be the result of a medical condition, pregnancy, etc. for certain people.

ii. You have to do this before you try to lose weight.

iii. Your physician and therapist can help you get started.

iv. Next, schedule a consultation with a dietitian to create a workout and food plan that you can stick to.

v. Seek their counsel and guidance on sustaining a healthy weight.

vi. To put an end to disordered eating, we must change our behaviour. Thus, eating problem behaviours will be discussed during therapy.

vii.   As a critical next step, your treatment team will attempt to identify any emotional or psychological issues that may be at the root of your binge-eating activity.

viii.   In addition to treating the behavioural and psychological components that contribute to the disease, it's vital to identify and treat any co-occurring disorders you may have.

ix.   Many people who suffer from binge eating also struggle with one or more other disorders in addition to the eating problem mentioned previously.

x.   Maintain a healthy diet and engage in regular exercise. By taking these steps, you can protect your heart and lower your chance of developing heart disease.

xi.   Speak with a doctor or dietitian for guidance on healthy eating and safe exercise.

xii.   You could also need medication to decrease your blood pressure, cholesterol, and blood sugar.

Cognitive behavioural therapy (CBT) is the primary and most effective treatment for conditions like depression, anxiety disorders, and binge eating.

Chapter Nine

How Does CBT Function?

In instances of severe anxiety or panic, cognitive behavioural therapy (CBT) teaches you to identify harmful habits and alter them, which may assist you in reframing your thoughts. It can also provide new coping mechanisms, like writing or meditation, for people who are struggling with addiction or hopelessness.

By giving depressed people the tools to challenge their negative thoughts and swap them out for more logical and upbeat ones, cognitive behavioural therapy (CBT) can aid in their recovery. Numerous other psychological conditions are also treated with CBT. In certain cases, it may be recommended to mix multiple therapeutic techniques for the greatest results.

Make an aid request. It might be difficult to quit binge eating on your own, particularly if there are underlying emotional problems at play. Working with a counsellor can help you discover the psychological factors, such as a negative body image, that contribute to binge eating.

Binge eating disorders require specialized care and treatment. Binge eating disorders pose a threat to an individual's mental, emotional, and physical well-being.

The complexity of binge eating disorder makes it imperative to have a multidisciplinary care team to competently manage this illness from hospitalization until discharge. This treatment may include individual and group therapy, dietary counselling, therapeutic meals, medical monitoring, and a host of other services. A person may require residential or acute care. At an intensive or residential care level, a patient's treatment team frequently includes a therapist, nutritionist, and medical professional. A person with binge eating disorder can achieve long-term recovery by receiving treatment from a team of professionals for all facets of the eating problem.

Chapter Ten

Why Can't I Stop Binge Eating?

You are not alone; millions of people worldwide suffer from overeating and binge eating, which are far more prevalent than you may think. Why, therefore, does it seem like you can never stop eating at times? Firstly, it would be wise to visit your doctor if you're feeling extremely hungry. Though it's extremely rare, some metabolic and endocrine disorders might cause increased appetite. A few drugs may potentially affect one's appetite.

A strict diet is often the first step in a vicious cycle of compulsive overeating for many people. It is difficult to break the habit of binge eating when you try to stop since you end up doing it again. It will be difficult to stick to a diet if you do so because you are self-conscious about your weight or size, particularly if you turn to food as a coping mechanism. The restrictions are reinstated after you eventually lose them and overindulge in "forbidden" foods, which causes shame and guilt.

Getting out of the cycle could be difficult. Binge eating may be the result of negative feelings such as stress, worry, or despair. Nevertheless, the comfort that eating may bring is fleeting, and following binge eating episodes, individuals may feel ashamed, guilty, and upset. But what is already seductive, soothing, and comforting just gets more seductive when it is prohibited.

Chapter Eleven

Individualized Objectives to Avoid Binge Eating Disorders

When was the last time you ate so much that you were completely satisfied? Were you celebrating a friend's birthday? Were you eating a huge cake? Thanksgiving dinner mostly consists of turkey and sweet potatoes, or maybe it was just you and the dog at home after a difficult day. If you gave yourself a stomachache, you must have felt bad about yourself afterwards. Or did you experience regret or guilt?

It is typical to periodically consume excessively. Emotional consumption is also permissible. Food has been utilized to nourish and reward every single infant since the time of creation. Food, thus, influences our human nature and feelings.

Some folks just eat too much because it's their habit, like when they regularly curl up with a bag of chips in front of the TV at night. It all started with this habit. That often, though, is the result of deeper emotional problems. Having a negative body image could be a major contributing factor.

Avoid Calling Yourself Wrong: You should understand that you are not a horrible person who is doing badly; rather, you are a good person who was created good. If you identify and label yourself as a terrible person, it becomes a self-fulfilling prophecy, and the cycle continues.

Maintain Yourself with Healthy Habits of Life: A physically fit, relaxed, and well-rested person is better equipped to manage life's inevitable curveballs. However, when you're already exhausted and overworked, even a small setback could send you spinning and into the refrigerator. When you exercise and get enough sleep, you can prevent binge eating, and other lifestyle decisions.

Don't Judge certain Foods Based on Moral Principles: All that God has created is for human consumption, yet we still need to choose the right amount and time to eat each meal.

<u>Timetable Frequent Workout</u>: Engaging in physical activity can significantly reduce stress and improve your attitude and energy levels. The natural mood-boosting effects of exercise can help reduce the likelihood of emotional eating.

<u>Always Stop and Think Things Through</u>: Whenever you have the want to eat, stop and think about if you are truly hungry. It is more important to think about why you want to eat than it is to focus on what to eat. If you use food as a coping strategy, it's important to bring your attention back to your body because you might not recognize the cues your body gives you to indicate whether you are satisfied or hungry.

<u>Reduce Tension</u>: One of the most important aspects of controlling binge eating is to identify healthy substitutes for utilizing food as a coping mechanism for stress and other intense emotions. These could include exercise, meditation, and sensory-relaxation approaches.

<u>Modify Your Environment</u>: A change in your environment can provide you the chance to select something that has greater meaning and assist you in refocusing on your efforts.

Relationship Building: Social connections and the relationships you have with the people you care about are crucial. You are more prone to succumb to stimuli that lead to binge eating if you lack a solid support network. Speak with someone, even if they're not a professional.

Manage Your Appetite: Refusing to eat certain meals may cause you to overindulge later. Even if you don't, give yourself permission to indulge in a small amount if you genuinely crave it.

Give Up Restrictive Diets: "There are benefits and drawbacks to both overindulging and eating in moderation. Just as deprivation can exacerbate overeating, restriction can also result in tension, fury, or worry.

Obtain Enough Sleep Every Night: Your body craves sugary foods that will give you a quick energy boost when you don't get enough sleep. Sleep deprivation can also lead to the onset of a food addiction. Your mood will improve, your appetite will be better controlled, and your cravings for food will decrease if you get enough sleep.

How to Stop Binge Eating: Although a lot of people have trouble with it, the tendency to binge eat can be somewhat broken. Long-term "management" or "coping" with binge eating is not required. No matter how often or how long you have been binge eating, there is a great deal of hope for total freedom from this practice.

Rather than excessive eating or simply eating for the purpose of eating, binge eating is caused by a few fundamental misconceptions about how our thoughts, feelings, and behaviours actually work. Understanding yourself, your thoughts, feelings, and the nature of binge eating from the inside out is essential to achieving liberation.

However, as was previously said, binge-eating disorder (BED), is a serious eating problem that can be cured, and it is characterized by recurrent episodes of extremely high food consumption (usually quite rapidly and to the extent of discomfort). It is the most common eating disorder in the United States.

BED is among the most recent eating disorders to be formally recognized in the DSM-5. Prior to the most recent modification in 2013, BED was classified as an EDNOS subtype. It is currently known as OSFED, which stands for "other specified feeding and eating disorder." An eating disorder is diagnosed in those who do not fit the diagnostic criteria for any other OSFED. The change is essential because, without a DSM diagnosis, some insurance companies won't cover treatment for eating disorders.

The Diagnostic and Statistical Manual of Mental Disorders (DSM) is the gold standard for diagnosing mental illnesses and is used by medical practitioners throughout the majority of the world, including the United States. The DSM contains descriptions, symptoms, and further diagnostic standards for mental illnesses.

Additional medical interventions:

     i.   Cognitive behavioural therapy and other counselling techniques are used to treat binge eating disorders in order to teach patients how to follow a more regular, healthy eating schedule and to interrupt their binge eating behaviour.

ii.   Therapy and medication intended to address underlying issues can also be useful forms of treatment. The long-term efficacy of anti-obesity drugs and bariatric surgery in lowering obesity and hunger is questionable, making them more contentious than other treatments.

iii.   To summarize, a person with binge eating disorder will eat a lot of food in a short amount of time, at least once a week for several months. The disease is frequently linked to further underlying mental health issues or a preexisting negative body image belief. Effective treatment options for underlying issues include medication and therapy.

Chapter Twelve

Is it possible to stop binge-eating?

It is feasible, yes. I'll respond to your question from a spiritual and religious perspective. As a believer and someone who puts their trust in God's word, nothing is impossible for God. In reality, with God's help and the inner spirit of Jesus, who gives us the ability to accomplish anything, there is no addiction that cannot be overcome.

By this, I mean that in order to overcome any obstacle in life, no matter how little or potentially fatal, one must have faith in the unchangeable and achievable nature of God's word. On the other hand, persistence is necessary to succeed in any endeavour. It is concentrated on achieving a victorious conclusion through intense prayer and fasting. Intermittent fasting, if one is committed to it, can help someone recover from binge eating disorders.

Many professionals advised those who had long-term binge eating disorders to accept that they would always suffer from the disorder and to be ready for the habit to recur anytime they felt overwhelmed or worried. A number of these individuals talked about how the power of the Holy Spirit's indwelling enabled them to overcome binge eating disorders.

Now, the majority of people who binge eat do so because they feel powerless to stop eating. And usually it happens quickly, quickly, and until you're uncomfortable, even if you're not hungry, alone, and usually emotional - disturbed, agitated, depressed, etc., because you find yourself in it once more.

Taking daily stock of oneself is the finest practice to recommend. Observe how you feel following a meal. Take note of it for yourself and see what occurs when you switch to a different dish after taking a few bites of this one.

Has the change made it stronger? What is the duration of its strength? When does it begin to decline? You can use this type of research as a technique to help you stay mindful and in the moment as you eat. And that's the intention.

Therapy, either with or without medication, is the primary treatment for binge eating disorder.

Dialectical behaviour therapy for eating disorders, guided self-help, cognitive behaviour therapy, and interpersonal therapy are the evidence-based therapies for borderline eating disorder (BED). Binge-eating that arises from overly rigorous diet regimens and obsessive attention to one's body image is addressed by cognitive behavioral therapy. Therefore, the therapy improves your perception of yourself and promotes healthier eating habits. You can perform this type of therapy on your own without a therapist by using guided self-help in cognitive behaviour therapy.

The Diagnostic and Statistical Manual of Mental Disorders is often known as the DSM. Most medical practitioners in the United States and the majority of other countries use it. The DSM provides guidelines, symptoms, and other information to aid in the diagnosis of mental illnesses.

The DSM now recognizes binge eating as a legitimate diagnosis category. It is characterized by recurrent episodes of overeating or bingeing, as well as a lack of control because the person keeps bingeing despite wanting to stop and taking practical steps to do so, but they end up repeating the same behaviour.

Furthermore, remember that those who have a disordered connection with food and disordered eating behaviours in general are the focus of this, not just those with officially diagnosed eating disorders. If it's required, I can advise you to get diagnosed. However, I think a lot of us who are affected by diet culture fall somewhere along the spectrum of having a disordered relationship with food.

Conclusion

The general public as well as people who frequently turn to overeating as a coping strategy are the target audience for this book. Everyone overeats periodically, but binge eating goes beyond simple overindulgence, such as during Thanksgiving or other formal dinners. It's extreme and starts happening frequently.

This book studied the definition, causes, and symptoms of binge eating, as well as everything related to it. It is anticipated that it would help someone kick the habit of binge eating.